D1765472

Items should be returned on or before the last date shown below. Items not already requested by other borrowers may be renewed in person, in writing or by telephone. To renew, please quote the number on the barcode label. To renew online a PIN is required. This can be requested at your local library.
Renew online @ **www.dublincitypubliclibraries.ie**
Fines charged for overdue items will include postage incurred in recovery. Damage to or loss of items will be charged to the borrower.

ed.

aged.

ptoms,
ids,
aging

Leabharlanna Poiblí Chathair Bhaile Átha Cliath
Dublin City Public Libraries

Baile Átha Cliath
Dublin City

Ráth Eanaigh
Raheny Branch
Tel: 8315521

Date Due	Date Due	Date Due

1

Published by IMB Publishing 2014

Table of Contents

Table of Contents

Table of Contents

Table of Contents

Foreword

Tarsal tunnel syndrome is a rare condition that can prove hard to diagnose. Some of the symptoms can be similar to many other painful foot disorders, which can make it difficult to identify and hard to treat.

However, with a proper understanding of the causes of tarsal tunnel syndrome and of the treatments available, patients can play an active role in understanding their condition and in finding how to manage it.

As medical research continues into tarsal tunnel syndrome, there will, in the future, be more medical interventions to help successfully treat this type of nerve entrapment.

In the meantime, this book brings together the most commonly used medical techniques that are employed to manage this condition, along with alternative, natural methods that can be used to aid the patients recovery.

This book will help empower patients to take charge of their condition and learn to overcome the difficulties that this painful nerve compression can cause.

Introduction

Heel pain can be a disabling condition for many people and it can be among the most difficult types of pain to target, especially when conventional treatments fail.

In this book, you'll learn how to cope with a specific type of heel pain called tarsal tunnel syndrome. As well as explaining exactly what tarsal tunnel syndrome is, the book will also detail how to best manage the pain caused by this condition and the available treatments and aids that can help the reader to make this condition more manageable.

The reader will also find some of the best alternative therapies to help treat this type of heel pain and they will also discover:

- Effective exercises to help reduce pain
- Stretches to help limit the tightness around the affected area
- Orthotics and aids that can ease the discomfort
- Pain management
- Surgical options
- Forums where readers can share their experiences
- Tips to speed rehabilitation time
- And how this condition is diagnosed

Tarsal tunnel syndrome is a complex condition to treat, however, by providing practical advice and detailing the best treatments available, this book can help the reader to determine an action plan so they can find ways to help themselves.

The aim of this book is to provide a complete guide to present the reader with the available options to help get them back to their everyday activities that they used to enjoy and to allow them to find effective treatments and management tools to make life with their heel pain much better.

The book will also examine some of the other causes of heel pain and explain what the reader can do to help manage their discomfort.

Heel Pain – Statistics

Discomfort in the heel region of the foot is perhaps one of the most common causes of foot pain. According to the statistics from the British Columbia Podiatric Medical Association, 15% of the patients who consult a podiatrist do so because they are experiencing some form of heel pain.

The majority of patients reporting this type of discomfort are usually diagnosed with common disorders such as plantar fasciitis or an Achilles tendon problem; the statistics from British Columbia Podiatric Medical Association show that the most common cause of heel pain is plantar fasciitis, with more than 70% of patients seeking treatment for this condition.

The figures also show that the majority of people with plantar fasciitis or heel pain will get better without the need for any form of surgical intervention.

In addition, statistics indicate that plantar fasciitis and heel spurs are most often seen in female patients. Although these are among the most common causes of discomfort in the heel region, there are many other different reasons for heel pain and some of the most common will be explored in the book.

However, a lesser known condition called tarsal tunnel syndrome could also be the cause of heel pain, and its symptoms can sometimes mimic that of plantar fasciitis or Achilles tendonitis, making the condition harder to diagnose and even more difficult to treat. Sports injuries or an inflamed tendon can also lead to the development of tarsal tunnel syndrome.

Tarsal tunnel syndrome is a relatively rare condition and can be hard to manage, but this book will help you to create a detailed treatment plan using both medical and natural alternatives to ease your pain.

As you read on, you'll learn how to treat tarsal tunnel syndrome and you might even discover how to cure it.

Chapter 1) Tarsal Tunnel Syndrome explained

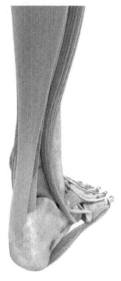

1) What is Tarsal Tunnel Syndrome?

Mary Aspinwall is the editor of The Clinical Medical Guide, author of the Basic Guide to Homeopathy, and the designer of the www.homepathyworld.com/s bestselling kits.

In the next section, Mary Aspinwall explains what tarsal tunnel syndrome is and some of the causes of it.

Tarsal tunnel syndrome occurs when there is a compression of the tibial nerve as it passes through the tarsal tunnel. It is characterized by a range of symptoms, including tingling, electric shock-like sensations, radiating pains, burning, chilliness, numbness, "pins and needles", cramping, heightened sensitivity and a build-up of fluid in the foot.

2) Tarsal tunnel syndrome - causes

Over exertion and standing for lengthly periods can make these symptoms worse, which is why it is often an occupational hazard and also affects athletes. There are many possible causes for TTS and it is always helpful to know the aetiology, as this will have an impact on how you deal with it.

For instance, a pinched lumbar or sacral nerve can lead to TTS and this would be best addressed by a chiropractor or an osteopath. Another factor is having flat feet, where orthotics may be needed. If the complaint came on after taking a new pharmaceutical drug, then it could be idiopathic (a side effect of the medication.)

A common cause of TTS is injury, such as a broken or sprained ankle or a repetitive strain type injury that has affected the joint, muscles or tendons.

3) Other symptoms of Tarsal Tunnel Syndrome

Further symptoms of tarsal tunnel syndrome include:

–   Muscle atrophy
–   Ankle pain
–   Pain in the toes
–   Unusual sensations in the feet and legs
–   Swelling in the ankle

4) Diagnosis of Tarsal Tunnel Syndrome

The first step towards diagnosing your condition should be a visit to your family doctor. Once you have described the symptoms, then your GP should be able to make a diagnosis. However, further tests might be required to confirm that you do indeed have tarsal tunnel syndrome.

There are several methods of confirming the diagnosis of this complex nerve condition.

In recent years a new test was devised, as it was felt that some of the other examinations for tarsal tunnel syndrome weren't reliable. The new test, which was devised by surgeons from the Department of Orthopedic Surgery, Osaka Medical College, is called the dorsiflexion-eversion test.

During the dorsiflexion-eversion examination, the consultant or physician will dorsiflex the foot into its maximum position while the foot is also everted. The doctor will also hold the metatarsophalangeal joints in the maximum dorsiflexed position for up to ten seconds.

The Tinel Test is another way of diagnosing the condition. In this test, the back of the ankle is tapped. If this produces a shooting pain, or other types of nerve pain, then it is considered a sign that the patient does have tarsal tunnel syndrome.

Musculoskeletal ultrasound is becoming an increasingly popular way to help this type of nerve compression. This form of diagnostic test can be especially useful for patients suffering from neuropathic pain if it has not been possible to confirm a definitive diagnosis any other way.

Musculoskeletal ultrasound, or MSUS, as it is sometimes known, can give a quicker and more accurate diagnosis for patients, but isn't always commonly used.

5) Tarsal Tunnel Syndrome – MRI Scan

Carrying out an MRI scan can give a much better idea of what is going on inside the tarsal tunnel, and how the nerves are affected. An MRI scan can also help determine whether there are other factors contributing to the condition, such as a growth or scar tissue.

6) Nerve Conduction Studies

Nerve Conduction Studies are sometimes carried out to see how well the nerves are firing. In studies, patients who underwent a nerve conduction test were found to have abnormal sensory nerve conduction. When the sensory nerves are affected, this will give rise to symptoms such as shooting pains, feelings of electrical shocks, etc., which are symptoms that are often associated with tarsal tunnel syndrome.

Research studies have confirmed that Nerve Conduction Studies are an effective way of diagnosing this form of nerve entrapment.

7) Tarsal Tunnel Syndrome – EMG

An EMG is an effective means of identifying any abnormalities that occur in the electric activity that control the muscles; an EMG is often used to diagnose or confirm diagnosis of tarsal tunnel syndrome. It is also used to diagnose other types of neuropathy and to diagnose other nerve conditions.

8) Tarsal Tunnel Syndrome – Different terms and what they mean

When it comes to tarsal tunnel syndrome, your consultant or GP might make reference to several terms that you might not be familiar with. These terms can often be confusing and make it even more difficult to understand the condition, so detailed in the next section is some of these terms along with an explanation of what they mean.

Bilateral Tarsal Tunnel Syndrome

This simply means that tarsal tunnel syndrome has affected both sides of the body. Pain and discomfort, along with other symptoms of the condition will be experienced in both feet.

Medial tarsal tunnel syndrome

The condition might also be referred to as medial tarsal tunnel syndrome. It is the same thing and refers to the compression of the medial nerve.

Posterior tarsal tunnel syndrome

Tarsal tunnel syndrome might also be called posterior tarsal tunnel syndrome. This is simply a way of describing the entrapment of the posterior tibial nerve.

Distal tarsal tunnel syndrome

This refers to the compression of the lateral plantar nerve.

Anterior tarsal tunnel syndrome

Anterior tarsal tunnel syndrome is a much more rare condition that refers to the compression of the deep peroneal nerve or the branches of the peroneal nerve.

9) Tarsal tunnel syndrome recovery time

Once a nerve becomes damaged, the patient will likely find that it will take a relatively long time to heal. Nerves have a tendency to repair slowly, and it could be some months before a patient begins to show any improvement.

Recovery time will also be related to the cause of the tarsal tunnel syndrome; unless the underlying cause is addressed, then it is going to be extremely difficult to affect a cure for your symptoms.

10) Causes of Tarsal Tunnel Syndrome

The cause of tarsal tunnel syndrome can sometimes be hard to determine. However, it is often associated with diabetic patients and with arthritis.

Tarsal tunnel syndrome can also be caused by injury or trauma, or sometimes a growth.

Poor Biomechanics can also play a role in the development of this painful nerve compression.

Sometimes, the cause of tarsal tunnel syndrome remains a mystery in some patients and why a patient has developed this condition can't always be explained.

11) Treatment for Tarsal Tunnel Syndrome

In the early stages of the nerve entrapment, it is likely that a more conservative approach to treating the condition will be adopted. If the TTS proves difficult to treat, and the symptoms seriously begin to impair a patient's quality of life, then it may become necessary to consider surgery to reduce the compression/entrapment of the nerve to help relieve the symptoms.

An anti-inflammatory will often be prescribed in the early stages to help reduce pain, swelling and inflammation surrounding the tarsal tunnel. It might also be suggested that the patient ices the affected area to help reduce pain and inflammation.

Steroid injections might be suggested, and it is also likely that the patient will be advised to wear insoles or a brace to help counter issues, such as flat feet and pronation, that can contribute to tarsal tunnel syndrome.

Medication to alleviate the painful nerve sensations are also likely to be prescribed. Medications commonly suggested to help manage this condition include Neurontin, Lyrica and Lidocaine. Neurontin and Lyrica are known to reduce spasms, and Lidocaine is used as a form of topical pain relief.

Anti-depressants might also be given, as some forms of the medication are often used to help reduce nerve pain.

All of the above medicines can be a highly effective way of helping to manage the discomfort associated with tarsal tunnel syndrome.

Patients will also be advised to rest the affected area and patients will often be forced to take some time out from their usual activities if the pain caused by tarsal tunnel syndrome makes it too difficult to continue as normal.

12) Surgery for tarsal tunnel treatment

If the symptoms of tarsal tunnel syndrome remain, and all conventional treatments have been tried, yet there is still no significant improvement of the discomfort, then it is possible that surgery will be needed to release the compression in the tarsal tunnel area.

Tarsal tunnel syndrome surgery will act to decompress the flexor retinaculum and the tibial nerve will be released. The surgery is uncomplicated and it is usually carried out as a day case. However, if you have an underlying medical condition, such as diabetes, then it might be necessary to stay in for an extra day to ensure that the blood sugar stabilises afterwards.

18

The surgery works by making a cut into the tibial nerve, and the lateral and distal nerves will also be decompressed during the surgery. Once the nerve compression has been released, the patient should begin to notice a relief from the symptoms once they have recovered from the surgery.

The surgery does have a high success rate, and the surgery is considered as a largely safe procedure. However, some patients can develop complications following this type of surgery and the symptoms could then worsen. This is something to consider before the surgery, and all types of conservative treatments should have been tried first. If you are considering this type of surgery, discuss all possible outcomes of the operation first.

In the case of diabetic patients undergoing surgery, they will usually be advised to have breakfast as normal and then to go into the hospital ready for the surgery. Depending on the time of the surgery, a diabetic patient might be put on a glucose drip to maintain the blood sugars, which will be monitored carefully. Once the patient feels like eating again after the surgery, the drip will then be removed.

Anaesthetic

If a patient doesn't tolerate anaesthetic well, there are ways of avoiding undergoing a general anaesthetic, such as an epidural. Discuss your options with your surgical team.

After Care

The patient might be prescribed antibiotics after the surgery in order to keep the site clean and free from infection, and the patient will have to return to hospital to have the stitches removed. If someone is prone to blood clotting, then they would usually be given anti-clotting injections to help thin the blood while they are immobile.

13) Tarsal tunnel syndrome - physical therapy

Once the surgery is over and you are out of the cast, then the recovery can really begin. In the UK, patients will usually be referred to a physio, who will see them at their local hospital. The referrals can sometimes take a little while, so in the meantime, follow your surgeon's advice about exercise and rehabilitation. Appointments will often be every two-three weeks and once you have recovered sufficiently; you'll be discharged from the physio department.

A physiotherapist can offer specific advice to help patients get back on their feet, regain their mobility, and rebuild any muscles that might have atrophied while the leg was in a cast.

The therapist will help design a plan to address the patient's personal needs and act to address any problems with your mobility that you might be experiencing after surgery. For instance, if you have lost a lot of muscle while your leg was in a cast, then they will give you strengthening exercises to help rebuild them. The physio might also recommend exercises to help improve balance, as atrophied muscles can make it difficult to regain balance after surgery.

Your physio will also be able to best advise you on when it will be safe to start participating in your favourite activities and exercises again, as well as offer advice on how to avoid a reoccurrence in the future.

Make the most of your time with the physio and make sure that you explain all of the problems you have been experiencing after surgery so that they can properly help you. It is a good idea to write down any symptoms or questions that you might have following the surgery so that you don't forget to ask them while at the appointment.

If you are seeing an NHS physiotherapist then some areas have a limit on how many sessions you can have. In this case, see if you can find an affordable private therapist if you still feel that you need help with your recovery.

There is no need for a referral to go to a sports injury clinic and they can often see a patient within 24-48 hours, and this may also be a preferred method for some patients, as you can get appointment times that suit you.

Appointments can cost from £35-40 for a 30 minute session; details on how to find a sports injury clinic near you are detailed in the back of the book.

Chapter 2) Exercises for Tarsal Tunnel Syndrome

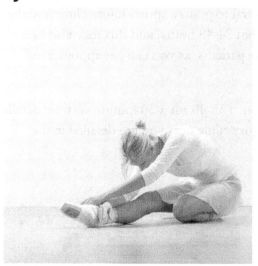

Exercise can be extremely beneficial for patients with tarsal tunnel syndrome. Although exercise in itself won't help cure the condition, it can help to reduce some of the symptoms.

If the compression of the nerve has been caused by inflammation, then care should be taken before adopting an exercise programme, as exercise could make the inflammation worse to begin with, especially if you are carrying out repetitive actions.

Maintaining a regular exercise programme will help to stop muscles from atrophying while you are inactive, however, you might need to change your exercise programme while you recover to ensure you that don't make the pain worse.

Exercise will also help to boost the circulation. Good circulation plays an essential role in helping the nerves to heal; poor circulation can cause symptoms such as tingling to feel worse.

When deciding on an exercise plan while you recover from tarsal tunnel syndrome, you should choose something that will help to length and strengthen the lower leg muscles and ankles.

The areas you'll specifically want to work on include the tendons in and around your ankle, the calf muscles and the shin muscles. If your balance has been affected, if you have flat feet, or if you have feet that pronate when you walk then you can also benefit from doing exercises to help reduce pronation and that will strengthen the arches.

Stretches should be balanced out with strengthening exercises. Perhaps experiment with a few different exercises first so that you can monitor which ones work for you and which exercises might make the symptoms worse.

If you haven't exercised for a while, then non-weight bearing exercises are a good place to start. Swimming is a great option for many people and is ideal during the rehabilitation period. Swimming is also good for patients with arthritis, as it is gentle on the joints.

Regular walking will help to keep the muscles toned, but patients should not exercise to the point of discomfort and should only do as much as they can do without worsening the symptoms.

Gentle exercises using light weights will help to keep the muscles built up, but be careful not to do many repetitions or you risk causing inflammation in the already sore area.

Before beginning any extra exercise, there are a few notes of caution. First, speak to your doctor as only they can tell you which

23

activities will be most beneficial and the areas that you need to work on most. They can also advise if they think any of the exercises might cause further irritation.

Moreover, proper footwear and orthotics are essential for giving your feet some extra protection while you exercise. Wearing a sports shoe designed to properly protect the foot, and with gel cushioning to help take the stress off of your sore heel, is vital for when you exercise. There is a chapter on suggested footwear later on in the book and you'll find a list of suppliers at the back.

Listed in the next section of this chapter are some exercises to help stretch and strengthen the lower leg muscles and ankles. Please note it is important to consult with your doctor first before doing these exercises as I don't know your medical history.

Exercises for Stretching and Strength

1) Ankle Stretch

Directions:

Sit with your feet straight out in front of you. Use a belt or an exercise band, hook it around both ankles and then push against the belt or band so you are pointing your feet as far as they will go.

Once you have pointed your feet as far as they will comfortably go, then bring them up towards you, flexing them as far as you can – the aim should be a 90 degree angle, but if you have limited movement around the ankle area then this might not be possible.

2) Ankle Circles

Directions:

Lie on your back with one knee bent and the other leg out straight. Bring your straight leg into your chest and hook your hands under your knee. Circle your ankle five times to the left and then five times to the right.

3) Ankle Circles – Alternative

Directions:

Sit up straight in a chair with both feet on the ground. Lift one foot off the floor and circle your ankle. Begin the circles as small as possible and as the ankle joint warms up, slowly increase the size of the circles. Keep repeating the circles, taking your ankle through its complete range of motion. Continue this until your ankle tires, then repeat on the other side. Stop if this exercise causes any pain.

4) Calf Stretch

Stretching your calf will help to improve range of motion in the ankle area. For a gentle calf stretch, sit up straight on a chair or on the edge of a bed. Hook an exercise strap or a belt underneath your arches. Holding the strap in your hand pull it until your feet lift off the ground and you feel a light stretch in the calf region.

The calves can also be stretched by facing the wall, lining up the front foot against the wall and stepping back with the other leg. Just take a small step back to get a light stretch. Bend your knee when you stretch to make it more comfortable if you need to, and take care with this stretch if you feel pain in your heel.

Repeat the stretch three times each side and hold each position for 10-15 seconds, but come out of the move before then if you begin to feel discomfort.

5) Calf Raises

Calf raises are one of the best exercises for helping to keep the calf muscles strong.

Directions:

To do this exercise, hold on to a sturdy object and wrap your left foot around your right leg. Rise up onto the toes of your right foot, hold for a few seconds, and then lower back down.

The exercise should be continued for as many repetitions as are comfortable and then repeated on the other side.

6) Soleus Stretch

The Soleus muscle runs from below the knee and into the heel. The Soleus is used in everyday actions such as walking and standing. It is not often that this muscle gets much of a stretch, but as it is so closely situated to the calf, it is important to focus on this area, too.

Directions:

Place one foot so that it is touching the wall. The other foot should be behind you and bent at the knee. Hold this stretch for up to thirty seconds and then repeat the move on the other side. This exercise should be repeated three times on each leg, however, if you find this stretch makes the back of your knee sore, reduce the amount of times you do this exercise.

7) Shin Exerciser

This exercise will strengthen the shin and the calf area. By building up the muscle in the lower leg, it will make it easier to lift your foot when you walk.

The better able you are to lift your foot, the less your foot will pronate, so exercising this area can be beneficial to patients who have developed tarsal tunnel syndrome due to the compression caused by the foot pronating.

Directions:

Sit up straight with your feet flat on the floor. Raise your heels and then tap your toes. Keep alternating the movements for 10-20 repetitions – less if you feel any pain.

Arch Exercises

Strengthening the arch can help provide greater stability to the foot and ankle when you are walking, thus reducing pronation and the subsequent overuse of the tendons that often occurs when your foot rolls inward.

If your feet roll inwards when you walk, try to gently push your feet towards the outside as you move. The aim should be so that your heel strikes the ground at the center, rather than on the outside of the foot.

Doing this will reduce the strain on the muscles of the foot and can help to strengthen the arch as you walk; it can, over time, reduce pronation.

8) Arch Scrunch

The following exercise is designed to strengthen your arches.

Directions:

Sit up straight with your feet flat on the floor and scrunch your arch, making it appear higher. Hold for a few seconds and then release.

9) Towel Scrunch

Put a towel in front of you and use your toes to scrunch up the towel bit by bit, squeezing the arches as you do. Repeat this exercise as many times as is comfortable. This exercise is also suitable for people prone to ankle sprains.

10) Standing arch exercises

Stand with your feet close together then push your weight onto the outsides of your feet. Repeat this exercise up to 30 times.

Another way of helping to reduce pronation is by sitting with your feet out in front of you and resting them on the outer edges. You can stay in this position for as long as you find comfortable, but be careful not to hold it for too long or you risk the lower leg muscles tightening up and going into spasm.

Improving Balance

Lack of exercise, muscle atrophy, or a recent ankle injury, are all factors that can help contribute to poor balance. Poor balance leaves a person more prone to injury from falling and can also cause people to lose confidence in going out because of the fear of falling.

Some yoga poses are particularly beneficial for strengthening the arches of your feet and for improving balance, but none of the moves should be attempted without proper instruction.

Try Eagle, Tree or any of the standing poses that are common in yoga. These exercises will help improve balance as well as aiding concentration and focus. Just hold the moves for a few seconds to begin with and then increase as your balance improves. These exercises will also serve to improve the strength in the standing leg.

Yoga exercises, such as the Hero pose, also help to increase the range of motion in the feet and can help to make your feet more mobile; with regular practice your ankles will become more flexible.

This form of exercise is also beneficial for relaxing the muscles, reducing the pain caused by spasms, and helping to elongate tight, short muscles.

Many of the yoga poses will help stretch the lower leg and ankle area, which can be beneficial for patients with tarsal tunnel syndrome

11) One Leg Balance

Stand up straight and curl your left leg in towards your buttock or hold it just a few inches above the ground if this feels more comfortable. Hold for as long as comfortable and then switch to the other side.

Hold on to something supportive, such as a sturdy chair, if your balance needs some work. Don't be concerned if you wobble or sway from side to side to begin with; this will improve as time goes by and as you build strength.

This exercise is particularly good if you have just one side affected by tarsal tunnel syndrome, as the exercise helps to balance out uneven leg strength.

12) Meditation Pose

Sitting in meditation pose with your legs crossed in front of you can also be beneficial, as it rests your feet on the outer borders, taking some of the stress off the inner borders of your feet. Try doing this when your feet feel tired or sore, but don't hold the move for too long in case the muscles tighten up and go into spasm, as this will make the pain worse.

13) Squat Variation

This move was adapted after an Achilles injury. The aim with this move was to build up calf muscle, but to avoid putting too much strain onto the Achilles tendon.

Stand against the bed so that your lower legs are against the bed. Lower down to just above the bed and then rise back up, squeezing the buttock muscles as you do.

You should feel this exercise in the calves; this is one of the most effective ways of isolating them and working the muscles harder. Only do a few repetitions of these, as they are hard on the muscles and the aim is to avoid overworking the Achilles.

14) Seated Calf Raise

Sit up straight on a sturdy chair, a sofa, or a bed. Raise your feet until you feel the contraction in your calf. Repeat at least 10 times with the hands on the knees to provide some gentle resistance.

Next, lift your heels up until your feet are on tip toes and hold the move.

Remember to balance out any calf exercises you do with shin exercises. Muscles work in pairs, so if you work one muscle, you must exercise the opposing muscle or you'll risk creating an imbalance

15) Tibia Stretch

As you stretch the muscles of the back of the leg, it is important to also focus on the muscles at the front so that you don't create an imbalance between the muscles, which could lead to a tightening up of the shin muscles and make it difficult to lift your foot.

The Tibia anterior muscle is at the front of the lower leg and is essential for the dorsiflexion of your foot as you walk; it also helps to invert the foot

When your foot is held in plantar flexion or pointed position, this stretches the muscle down the front of the leg. To stretch this muscle you can sit with your legs straight out in front of you either on the bed or the floor. Point your toes until they touch the floor. You should feel this move in front of your leg. Repeat three times, but do fewer repetitions if it is making your muscles ache.

16) Alphabets

Alphabets are a simple, fun exercise that builds the arches as well as strengthening the ankles and improving balance.

In addition to being suitable for people with Achilles injuries, this is also good for people with plantar fasciitis or with ankles that have been weakened from sprains and strains.

Directions:

Sit on the edge of the bed. Sit far enough back so that your feet are off the floor. Draw the alphabet with your feet, one letter at a time,

31

ensuring that you take your ankle through the complete range of motion to get the most out of the exercise.

Repeat as many times as is comfortable.

17) Calf and Achilles stretch

Face the wall and stand with your toes against it. Step back with your right foot so that your heel is on the ground and also facing the wall. Next, lean forward using your arms to press into the wall and feel the stretch all the way down to the back of the leg. The stretch should be held for up to 30 seconds and then repeated on the left side.

Each stretch should be completed three times.

18) Alternative Calf Stretch

If you don't feel much of a stretch, this could be due to excessive tightness in the calves or Achilles. If this is the case, then push your weight onto the outer edges of your foot as you stretch. This should give a more powerful stretch, but you need to take care with this in case it is too much for the already vulnerable tendon area. The stretch should only be held for a short while; long enough to feel the effects but not so long that it causes pain.

19) Another Calf Stretch

Using a stair or step to support you, place your toes on the edge of the step and tilt your foot off the step so just the front part of your foot remains on it. This will give a much deeper stretch, but should be approached with caution if you are still recovering from injury.

By bending the back leg, it is possible to get a stretch in the muscles lower down, so you'll be able to target a tight Achilles tendon this way, too, but be careful not to put undue pressure on the tendon when you complete this stretch.

When completing any of the above exercises, ensure that they don't cause any undue pain and only do as many as you can comfortably manage.

If you feel any discomfort during any of the moves, then stop and start with low repetitions while you build up strength and flexibility and recover from your symptoms.

Chapter 3) Tarsal Tunnel Supports, Shoes and Braces

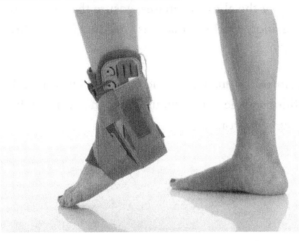

Wearing a support for the tarsal area can help to relieve some of the symptoms. They are especially useful if you are very active and need the additional protection and they might also be suggested for use after tarsal tunnel surgery to help provide comfort for the tarsal tunnel area as it heals.

Doctors might also suggest the use of a walking boot to help rest the foot and provide compression to the ankle region, which will help to ease some of the symptoms.

If inflammation contributes to your pain and discomfort and you find repetitive actions, such as walking or running, make the pain you feel worse, then you could also benefit from wearing a tarsal support either when you exercise or to provide additional protection when you plan on being more active.

Foot and Ankle Supports

Supports for the tarsal tunnel come in many different forms, so it a matter of finding out which one is best suited for your needs. For example, if you exercise a lot, then you'll want something that is durable as well as functional to allow you to engage in the kind of activities that you normally would without limiting your mobility or ability to exercise.

1) Swede 0- Tarsal

These supports provide additional protection to the ankle area, preventing it from rolling in or pronating. The support uses a stirrup design that protects both sides of the ankle and helps to stabilize the foot, stopping it from rolling in when you move.

2) Aircast A60 Ankle Cast

The Aircast A60 is rumoured to be worn by Wimbledon champion Andy Murray. These supports are designed to be lightweight while providing maximum support and comfort to the foot.

As well as being worn to help give support for patients with tarsal tunnel syndrome, they can also be worn by people recovering from fractures or people who suffer from ankle instability.

3) Power Ionics® Ankle Brace Support

These are made with bamboo charcoal fibre and will give warmth and compression to the affected area. They can also help to provide pain relief and they will help to aid circulation, too.

Ankle Sleeves

Ankle sleeves can also be useful for giving the foot and ankle some added stability. Listed below are details of some of the most popular brands. However, ankle sleeves might not be suitable for patients with circulation problems, so seek medical advice before purchasing and using one of these products.

4) Pro-Tec Ankle Support

Pro-Tec Ankle Support provides compression to the ankle, helping to reduce any swelling that might have occurred as a result of the tarsal tunnel syndrome. It also offers warmth to the area and will help to ease inflammation.

5) Silipos Malleolar Sleeve

The Silipos Malleolar Sleeve offers support to the front and back of the foot as well as giving the ankle protection. It has a gel cushioning for comfort and the sleeve will also provide some degree of compression to the ankle region.

6) Fs6 Compression Foot Sleeve

This sleeve offers six different support zones and has three levels of compression. It promotes oxygen and blood flow and can help speed up healing times for the injured foot.

This type of sleeve is particularly good for people who spend a lot of time on their feet and who have swelling in their foot or pain in the ankle region.

These are also beneficial for patients with plantar fasciitis; they can be worn all day and in sports shoes to give additional support while exercising.

Orthotics for tarsal tunnel syndrome

There's a huge range of orthotics available. However, there is a limit to how effective they can be, as the over-the-counter type of orthotics won't always provide the best support for your foot. In this case, it is best to visit one of the specialist clinics that make bespoke orthotics. Listed below are some orthotics that may be beneficial for patients with tarsal tunnel syndrome by helping to reduce pronation.

7) Sorbothane Sorbo-Pro Total Control

These insoles help to absorb shock and have additional support in the arch and ankle areas to help prevent the foot from pronating while in motion.

They are especially beneficial for people who participate in a lot of outdoor sports or do a lot of running.

8) Scholl Ortha Heel Insoles

These shoes are ideal for runners, as they have been designed to stop the foot from rolling from side to side while running, thus reducing the pronation that can contribute to conditions such as tarsal tunnel syndrome.

They also offer an additional layer of shock absorption and cushioning.

9) Sole Control Classic

The Sole Control Classic has a deep heel cup to help provide extra support for the heel region. They are helpful at reducing heel pain and can help to reduce pronation.

10) Dr. Scholl's Insoles Tri-Comfort Orthotics

These insoles give cushioning and protection, while being gentle on the feet.

They will act to reduce pain in both the heel and ball of the foot and can help to limit the feelings of fatigue that often come with standing on the feet all day.

11) Spenco Total Control

Some insoles can be extremely bulky, taking up a lot of room in the shoe making them uncomfortable to wear for a long period of time. Spenco Total Control is a slim fitting insole so does not have this problem.

As well as helping to reduce pronation, these insoles aid shock absorption, helping to prevent pain in the ankles, knees and hips that might occur as a result of too much stress on the foot.

The insoles also reduce pressure on the ankle and help to limit supination, or the rolling outwards of the foot, which can also case a number of foot injuries.

12) Healix Care Controltec

These insoles are made with bamboo and aim to keep the feet cool in the summer and warm in the winter. They come with a deep heel seat that is designed to prevent heel pain; the insoles also offer a greater stability for the ankle joint, preventing it from rolling inwards.

These insoles are firmer and more supportive than some other brands and are designed to help people with ankle and heel pain. They come with a gel heel to provide cushioning for the heel region and give metatarsal support for the comfort of the toes.

Shoes for Tarsal Tunnel Syndrome

Choosing the correct footwear is one way of helping to prevent the onset of tarsal tunnel syndrome. There are a range of shoes that come with a gel insert, which is especially helpful for patients with tarsal tunnel syndrome, as the gel will help to relieve any pressure in the heel area, thus reducing the compression of the nerve.

You should also ensure that the shoes you choose have enough support in them so that your ankle doesn't roll inwards when you move; this is extremely important if you do a lot of running or walking.

It is also vital to make sure that you choose the right shoe for the right sports. For example, trail running would require a completely different shoe than the ones worn for tennis. Each movement puts a different kind of strain on the foot and only by finding suitable footwear, can you find a way of compensating for it.

13) New Balance Basics

New Balance has a range of sports shoes that can be helpful for patients with tarsal tunnel syndrome. There is a choice of trainers that give either extra cushioning or additional stability, depending on which you need the most.

The trainers are available direct from the New Balance website. If you are outside the US and have difficulty obtaining them, then please refer to the shopping directory at the back of the book.

14) Asics Shoes

Asics Shoes are readily available through most sports shops and they are affordably priced. They have shoes that are designed to compensate for a whole range of foot maladies, including over pronation and poor stability.

Braces for Tarsal Tunnel Syndrome

Braces are helpful for supporting the foot to alleviate the pressure off the tarsal tunnel. They are most beneficial to patients that have problems with their feet, such as pronation.

Braces might also be used after surgery while the foot heals. They are also good for wearing during exercise, as they will help counter any weakness in the feet or problems with the gait that can contribute to overuse and inflammation of the foot, which can eventually lead to pain.

15) Gel Ankle Brace Sroufe Health Care Products

A gel brace will provide compression to the ankle to help reduce any swelling that might be present while also providing stability for the ankle. These braces can be frozen before use, but you'll need to take care if you have a lack of feeling in your feet and make sure that the cold doesn't burn your skin.

Socks and Stockings for Tarsal Tunnel Syndrome

Compression socks and stockings can help bring relief for patients with this condition. However, some experts advise against using compression in patients with neuropathy, so seek advice first.

Compression stockings are sometimes prescribed by doctors to help manage symptoms, and are often available on the NHS, depending on which area you live in.

16) Sigvaris Compression Socks

These socks are made from cotton so they are comfortable to wear. They have been designed so that they won't rub against the skin or cause it to chafe, which is important, especially if you have a lack of feeling in your foot or ankle, as it could become easily damaged without realising it.

17) Prolotex FIR

Prolotex FIR Socks can help to reduce pain and inflammation caused by tarsal tunnel syndrome. They can also help to increase the circulation, thus reducing some of the symptoms such as tingling and numbness. It might take up to six weeks before an improvement is noticed in the symptoms.

18) Daylong Compression Stockings

Daylong provides a range of compression stockings; they also supply ankle sleeves. If you have been prescribed compression stockings then they can also fill prescriptions for patients.

19) Better Life Healthcare

Better life Healthcare sells stockings that give a light to medium compression to the foot and lower leg. They provide stockings that can boost the circulation, provide healing support for soft tissue injuries, and reduce the chance of blood clots.

Chapter 4) Alternative Treatments for Tarsal Tunnel Syndrome

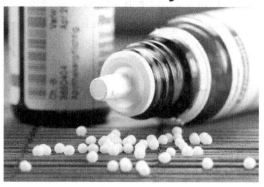

1) Homeopathy

Many people prefer the natural approach to their healthcare and rather than rely too heavily on medications, they like to try some of the natural alternatives.

These should only be used on a complimentary basis and should not be used at all without talking to your GP or consultant, especially if you are taking medication.

Care should also be taken with essential oils, especially if you are pregnant or suffer from epilepsy.

Homeopathy can play an important part in helping to alleviate some of the symptoms of tarsal tunnel syndrome. First, Mary Aspinwall explains the three most important rules about using homeopathy at home.

Three Golden rules for using homeopathy at home

Match your symptoms to the most similar remedy, having a homeopathy kit helps.

Take one dose. Only repeat if you had benefit, but later your symptoms returned.

Stick to a 30c potency (strength) for home use.

Injuries

The four most commonly needed injury remedies for TTS are **Arnica, Hypericum, Rhus tox** and **Ruta.**

Arnica is a great trauma remedy for bruising and shock. Use when the area feels weak, strained and swollen and the pain is stitching.

Hypericum is specific for injury to a nerve with shooting pains.

Rhus tox is a wonderful remedy for sprains in general, and is particularly helpful if you have a stinging pain in left heel.

Ruta is the go to remedy for damage to ligaments, tendons, the tendon sheath and the tarsal joint. The area feels bruised and there may also be paralysis of the tarsal joint.

Other factors that can reduce the space in the Tarsal Tunnel include:

Bone spurs

These can be relieved by supplementing with **Calc fluor 6x** (tissue cell salts) 4 pills, 3 times a day. Another homeopathic specific for bone spurs is **Hekla lava**.

<u>Ganglions</u>

Ganglions on flexor tendons respond well to **Ruta**.

Read the following descriptions to see if one of these remedies closely matches what you are experiencing.

Apis – electric shock through the toes, with redness, heat, swelling, stinging pains.

Arg nit – easy bending and straining of tarsal joint with violent, throbbing pain.

Belladonna – burning, tingling, itching, right sided, worse walking.

Hepar sulph – stiff, numb, drawing, burning.

Lachesis – drawing (pulling) pain, worse on the left side.

Ledum – swollen feet, rigid on waking, pain on stepping.

Lycopodium – pricking pain in the heel, sprained sensation, burning feet, soles are painful, worse for walking.

Merc viv – swelling, right foot, painful to touch.

Nat mur – bruised, gone to sleep sensation.

Sulph - Burning and itching in the soles. Swelling of the feet, - from warmth of the bed. Great heaviness in the feet, especially in the tarsal joints. Coldness and stiffness of the toes, with tingling of the tips.

2) Sports Massage

Many patients with tarsal tunnel syndrome find that a sports massage is beneficial to them. There are many types of massage that can be used and a sports therapist or a massage therapist will be able to advise which would be the best method for you.

Massage can help improve the range of motion of the foot and enhance mobility making it easy to walk. It can also help to reduce areas of tension in the foot and lower leg.

Studies have shown that cross friction massage can be especially beneficial to patients with tarsal tunnel syndrome.

3) Neuromuscular Massage

Neuromuscular massage will focus on trigger points and can be helpful at reducing pressure in the affected area as well as finding trigger points that might be contributing to the pain.

4) Orthobionomy

Orthbionomy is a little heard of technique that works to reduce pain that has been caused by stress or injury. The therapy is based on several healing techniques, including osteopathy.

Orthobionomy can enable the body to work better and improve the posture, allowing the body to move more freely and taking unnecessary stress off the joints.

This kind of therapy can also enhance the healing process. As well as being beneficial to patients with tarsal tunnel syndrome, it can also benefit patients with shoulder problems, migraines and difficulty sleeping.

It can be a useful method to help the body to counter stress, which can contribute to aches and pains throughout the body.

5) Muscle Energy Techniques

Muscle Energy is another form of massage that focuses on finding trigger points. Pressing on these trigger points can cause pain elsewhere throughout the body and reducing the pressure on these trigger points through massage can help relieve pain.

You'll find a link to a video demonstrating this technique on the resources page, so you can get a better idea of how it works.

6) Osteopathy

Osteopathy is a gentle, hands on technique that can help the body to function better, thus reducing pain when the person moves. As well as helping patients with lower leg discomfort, it can reduce joint pain and neck pain.

Osteopathy uses gentle stretching along with massage to help relieve pain throughout the body. This can be especially helpful if you have accumulated tension.

7) Aromatherapy

Aromatherapy won't cure tarsal tunnel syndrome, however, it can help to reduce some of the more uncomfortable symptoms, such as the tingling and burning sensations that are common in this disorder.

This form of therapy can prove effective in enabling the body to relax, thus reducing pain. It can also help to boost the circulation to the area and help the healing process.

Special aromatherapy blends are available for neuropathy and these are a good place to start. Frankincense and Myrrh are often used in a blend together to help reduce the symptoms, while peppermint oil has also been shown to be effective; lavender and camomile essential oils will help relax oversensitive nerves.

Oils should only be used once they have been properly blended with some carrier oil, as they are often too strong to be used directly against the skin without causing irritation. Coconut oil, Vitamin E oil and Sweet Almond oil all make an ideal base.

If you are unsure about the oils that would be most beneficial to you, seek the advice of an aroma therapist or buy a pre-blended mix that has been created to help alleviate the symptoms of nerve problems.

8)Chiropractor

A chiropractor can help to "adjust" the body, helping to relieve some of the tensions that might have built up. A chiropractor will often use a range of techniques to relieve the symptoms of tarsal tunnel syndrome, such as stretching or soft tissue therapy.

Chapter 5) Addressing the reasons behind your Tarsal Tunnel Syndrome

As detailed at the start of the book, tarsal tunnel syndrome can have many different causes. However, sometimes there is no known cause and the reason for it remains a mystery, this is often referred to as idiopathic tarsal tunnel syndrome, meaning that there is no recordable reason for the syndrome to have developed.

Here is a look at some of the most common triggers for tarsal tunnel syndrome and how you can make adjustments to try and counter them.

1) Tarsal Tunnel Syndrome and Running

Active people are more prone to tarsal tunnel syndrome. Actions such as running will cause an excess strain on the foot and the repetitive action of running can contribute to the overuse and inflammation that can play a role in the development of the condition.

The first step should be to ensure that you wear proper footwear. Shoes with a gel insole can help protect the foot in all of the right places and if you have a tendency towards pronation or if you have flat feet, then you'll need additional support, such as insoles and ankle sleeves or braces to help hold your foot in a better position. It is also worth consulting a sports therapist who will be able to suggest different taping methods in order to counter any problems with the position of your foot as you run.

Runners should also adopt a regular stretch programme to help relieve any tension in the muscles and weekly massage sessions are also a good idea.

48

A change of routine can also help to reduce some of the repetitive stress that would be caused by the running action. Creating a diverse routine is especially important if you tend to run every day, as your muscles need a rest from doing the same activity day in day out.

Runners are also prone to Achilles problems, which can lead to tarsal tunnel syndrome, so this is another area to be aware of.

2) Obesity

Being obese will put an additional strain on your feet and can cause problems with the biomechanics of how your feet work. This will produce an excess strain that can lead to inflammation, which in turn can contribute to the development of tarsal tunnel syndrome.

Being very overweight is also associated with joint pain, diabetes, some forms of cancer and heart disease – all extremely good reasons to change your lifestyle.

There is only one real answer to losing weight and that is to change your eating habits and begin an exercise programme. This is not something that should be done without the help of your doctor, so if this is a problem for you then see your GP, as they will be able to give you general diet advice and they can refer you to a dietician to help get you the tailored support that you would need in order to lose weight.

3) Diabetes

High levels of glucose will leave a diabetic patient more vulnerable to different types of neuropathy, including tarsal tunnel syndrome. When the glucose levels are high, this can lead to nerve damage, as well as many of the other complications that are associated with high glucose.

If your blood sugars are out of control, then speak to your diabetes nurse and ask for a referral to a dietician so that between them they can adjust your insulin dose and change your diet.

Also be aware that lifestyle, stress and a lack of sleep can contribute to poor glucose control, so these issues must be addressed too.

4) Low Thyroid

Low thyroid can leave a person vulnerable to tarsal tunnel and carpal tunnel syndrome. Low thyroid – or hypothyroidism – is common in diabetics; the symptoms include lack of energy, dry skin, low glucose levels and headaches.

Hypothyroidism is easily corrected by taking medication, so if any of these symptoms sound familiar, and you aren't already on thyroid medication, then ask your GP or consultant to run some tests if you aren't already tested on a regular basis for low thyroid levels.

5) Achilles Tendonitis

Achilles tendonitis can eventually lead to tarsal tunnel syndrome. Some of the causes behind tarsal tunnel syndrome, such as running or repetitive actions, poor biomechanics and pronation can also cause Achilles tendonitis.

In order to try and prevent tendonitis occurring, create a diverse exercise programme that does not include too much repetitive activity, use plenty of massage and stretch routines on the days when you don't exercise and wear proper sports shoes that are designed to protect your feet while you are running.

In addition, stop at the first signs of any feelings of discomfort in the Achilles area and seek special care to treat any of the symptoms of Achilles tendonitis as they occur; don't work through the pain and seek help at the first onset of discomfort.

6) Poor Circulation

Poor circulation can also be a contributor to tarsal tunnel syndrome. Bad circulation can also make feelings such as the tingling sensation experienced by sufferers worse.

To boost circulation, try some gentle exercise or if you are unable to keep active, perhaps try a circulation booster. These can help improve mobility as well as help to relieve swelling in the lower leg area, which will also act to alleviate some of the discomfort. However, they should not be used without consulting with a doctor first and they are not suitable for use by patients with blood clots in the lower area.

Take special care of your feet by making sure that they don't get too cold or too hot and choose socks that don't have elastic around the tops. Seam free socks are available and these are better for diabetics as they won't rub against the skin.

There are also nutritional aids that can help to boost the circulation. One supplement called Padma 28, a herbal supplement, can help boost the circulation and give relief to cold feet. This natural product is available in capsule form and can help relieve symptoms of poor circulation such as swelling, pain and cramps in the calf area.

7) Standing

Everyone knows the feeling of aching feet after they have been standing on their feet all day long and lengthly periods of being on your feet can be a contributor to tarsal tunnel syndrome.

If your job involves standing a lot, then wear comfortable shoes with a gel cushioning and wear gel insoles to help take the stress away from any pressure points of the feet.

Wear loose socks or compression stockings if swelling is a problem and try to change your actions at any available opportunity.

There are supplements and gels, such as antistax, that can help to improve circulation, make your feet feel lighter, and help reduce swelling.

8) Pronation

The excess strain caused to the feet by pronation can cause tarsal tunnel syndrome. Pronation can also contribute to other foot problems, such as plantar fasciitis and Achilles tendonitis. The stress placed on your feet when they pronate can also lead the way to pain and inflammation in the feet.

Footwear and supports are the most important aspects of managing pronation. Some gel based inserts can be very comforting to the feet and will help to provide cushioning and protection to the heel region.

Wear shoes that are supportive and that come with a gel cushioning to protect the heel area and to relieve pressure in the heel region.

Take care not to do anything too repetitive, as the poor biomechanics caused by pronation will easily lead to inflammation that can eventually lead to problems such as tarsal tunnel syndrome. In addition, always warm up before you exercise and stretch out afterwards.

9) Flat Feet

Having flat feet, or feet with no or little arch can also cause tarsal tunnel syndrome, due to the undue burden that having collapsed arches puts on the feet. This can lead to a compression of the tibial nerve, which can then lead to the symptoms of this condition.

Wearing orthotics can help to eliminate the tired, aching feeling that can sometimes be caused by flat feet and will take some of the stress away from the joints and the tendons.

Exercises can also be done to help strengthen the arches, helping to reduce some of pressure on the feet.

10) Injury

An injury to the foot, such as a sports injury or an ankle sprain, could pave the way to the development of tarsal tunnel syndrome. The swelling of the ankle after an injury could lead to a compression of the tibia nerves, leading to the symptoms commonly associated with this painful nerve compression.

Any type of trauma to the foot, especially an injury that causes swelling, could eventually lead to the development of tarsal tunnel syndrome.

11) Varicose Veins

Varicose veins are quite common and they can create pressure in the ankle region causing compression of the tibial nerve.

Varicose veins often don't require surgery unless they are causing a great deal of pain. Surgery might also be considered if the varicose veins have led to complications. They are common in people who stand a lot and compression stockings can be useful in helping to ease the symptoms.

12) Swelling of a tendon

Anything that causes swelling of the tendons in the foot might cause tarsal tunnel syndrome. If this is believed to be the case, scans can be carried out to see where the swelling is coming from and whether it is compressing the nerve.

13) Arthritis

Arthritis often causes swelling in the joints and this swelling could cause the nerve to become entrapped, producing the symptoms of tarsal tunnel syndrome.

In addition, arthritis can cause swelling and changes in the tendons, which again can cause an entrapment of the nerves.

A study carried out by the Rheumatology and Rehabilitation, Faculty of Medicine, Alexandria University, Egypt that involved motor nerve conduction tests, sensory nerve conduction tests, EMGs and ultrasonographic studies have confirmed that the syndrome is common in patients with rheumatoid arthritis.

14) Growth

A tumor or growth can cause the symptoms of tarsal tunnel syndrome to arise if the swelling causes a nerve impingement or if the tumor/growth compresses the tibial nerve.

This would only be in extremely rare cases; a growth or tumor can be detected by undergoing an MRI scan to see what is going on in the ankle/foot.

Whatever the cause of your heel pain, make sure that it is treated as quickly as possible so that it doesn't get any worse. Soft tissue injuries are difficult enough to treat at the best of times and leaving it too long will make the treatment times and rehabilitation process even longer.

See a sports therapist, a doctor or a physiotherapist if you have symptoms of any of the above conditions.

Chapter 6) Useful Vitamins, Minerals and Supplements

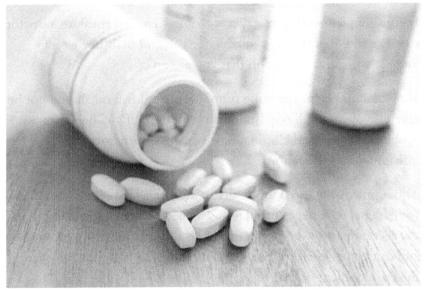

Additional nutritional support is helpful to the body to assist in the healing process. Vitamins are not enough to cure tarsal tunnel syndrome but they can go some way towards reducing some of the distressing symptoms, such as the tingling pains that are associated with nerve problems.

Other natural supplements can work to help reduce inflammation, which can in turn, help to reduce some of the swelling and pain if this is a problem for you.

While anti-inflammatories such as Ibuprofen are fine, when taken for a short time, they are believed to inhibit the healing process in some cases and they are not suitable for long-term use. For that reason, it might be preferable to find a natural approach that is less damaging to the body.

Natural anti-inflammatory products should not be taken alongside prescribed medication without speaking to your GP or Physician first.

Before supplementing your diet with any vitamins, speak to a doctor to make sure that they are suitable for you and that they won't interact with any medication that you are on.

Supplements such as evening primrose oil and fish oil should not be taken if you are on blood thinning medication, if you have any problems with blood clotting, or if you are on any form of anti-inflammatory medication.

The supplements listed in the first part of this chapter are beneficial for patients with nerve problems. The natural supplements listed in the second part of the chapter all have anti-inflammatory properties and can be beneficial to patients if inflammation has played a part in the development of their symptoms.

Vitamins and Minerals for Tarsal Tunnel Syndrome
1) B Complex

B complex vitamins are known to be beneficial to nerve health and a lack of some B vitamins, such as vitamin B12, can contribute to the tingling feelings experienced by people with neuropathy.

In addition, benfotiamine, a fat soluble form of vitamin B1 and methylcobalamin, a form of vitamin B12, have shown promise in reducing some of the symptoms of neuropathy.

2) Magnesium

Magnesium is a mineral known to relax the nerves and the muscles. It can help to alleviate symptoms such as cramps and muscle aches that can be associated with tarsal tunnel syndrome.

It can be taken as a supplement or applied as a cream or spray if you want to target the affected area directly. Epsom lotions are also available; these are made from Epsom salts and contain high levels of magnesium. This is useful for massaging in to sore areas of your ankle or heel.

Epsom salts can also be used to bathe the feet and help relax, sore aching muscles.

Natural Anti-Inflammatory Supplements
3) Evening Primrose Oil

If inflammation has contributed to the development of tarsal tunnel syndrome, it can be beneficial to supplement the diet with products known to reduce inflammation.

Evening Primrose Oil contains Omega 6, which is known to reduce inflammation. It can also help to limit the associated pain and swelling.

It is also believed to be beneficial for arthritis sufferers.

Evening Primrose Oil supplements should not be taken by patients on blood thinning drugs.

4) Alpha Lipoic Acid

Studies have shown alpha lipoic acid to improve the health of the nerves in the feet. It can help reduce the burning, stabbing and tingling feelings that often come as part of nerve entrapment or nerve damage.

It is helpful for patients with diabetic neuropathy and can lower blood sugar levels, however, it can also interact with some medications such as levothyroxine, so consult your GP before supplementing your diet.

5) Fish Oil

Fish Oil is another powerful but natural anti-inflammatory. Its Omega 3 oils are helpful for patients with joint pain and it is thought to promote heart health as well.

Fish Oil can also be taken in the form of cod liver oil. However, it should not be taken by patients on blood thinning drugs.

6) Ginger

Ginger is used by many as a remedy for inflammation. It is also believed to act as a mobility aid. Ginger supplements should be taken in their standardized form in order for it to be the most effective.

The herb is also known to act as a circulation booster and can be applied as an oil or used as a foot bath to help warm the feet.

7) Circumin

This spice has a number of medicinal uses, and can help to reduce inflammation and pain. It can also help to encourage the healing process and it's useful for those suffering from a sports injury such as tendonitis.

8) Boswellia

Boswellia is another natural anti-inflammatory. It can help to sooth pain and can be taken as a supplement or used as a cream to reduce pain and swelling.

Boswellia, or Frankincense, also works as an analgesic and can help to provide pain relief in nerve problems.

The cream is easy to apply to the affected area and will be absorbed quickly.

9) Pycnogenol

Pycnogenol acts as a powerful anti-oxidant and it is thought to have many health benefits. For instance, patients with diabetes might find this supplement – which is an extract of pine bark – effective as it is believed to help with retinopathy, a complication of long term diabetes that occurs in some patients.

Pycnogenol also has strong anti-inflammatory properties and could be helpful in the healing process.

Pycnogenol should not be taken by patients on corticosteroid drugs or immunosuppressant's.

10) Green Tea

Green tea contains high levels of anti-oxidants. It is thought to lower blood sugar levels, reduce blood pressure, protect the body from cancer, and lower cholesterol levels.

In addition, it works as an anti-inflammatory, which could help limit pain and swelling.

While many of the green tea products available contain caffeine, there are now some caffeine free products available if they are preferred, and there are also some flavoured versions for those that don't like the strong taste of the tea.

It can also be served with honey to add some natural sweetness to it.

11) Arnica

Arnica is well known for its healing properties and is often used for ankle sprains and bruising. In addition, arnica will act as a natural anti-inflammatory.

It should not be taken internally, but there are many creams and lotions available.

12) Ashwagandha

Studies have shown that ashwagandha can work as an anti-inflammatory. It can also contain high levels of antioxidants and can act as a rejuvenator. This herb is also believed to have a positive influence on the immune system.

It is possible that the herb has some influence on the thyroid gland, so care should be taken if you are on thyroid medication or if you have any problems with thyroid functioning.

13) Capsaicin

This herb has anti-inflammatory properties and it is a surprisingly effective pain reliever. It has also been proven to be effective in reducing discomfort in patients with neuropathy or other forms of nerve pain.

It is available in capsule form but for nerve pain, it is often more effective when applied as a cream. The cream can be applied to the affected area four times a day, but be careful of skin redness or irritation.

Diet

Adapting the diet so it contains plenty of foods beneficial to nerve health could also be helpful in your recovery from tarsal tunnel syndrome.

Supplementing the diet with vitamins and minerals is one way of improving the nutrition levels; however, it is also a good idea to give your body some of the extra nutrients it needs through diet.

An improved diet will also enable the body to be better able to cope with stress and will help boost energy and blood sugar levels to.

The nerves require good levels of essential vitamins such as B complex vitamins and minerals like magnesium to help nourish them and heal them.

A diet high in cereals and grains will contain good levels of B vitamins, which will be helpful for the nerves and the nervous system. B Vitamins are also found in pulses and lentils, liver and green vegetables.

Magnesium intake can be increased by eating green leafy vegetables, nuts and seeds, rice, yogurts and bananas.

Diet can also help to reduce inflammation naturally, and there are many foods that have an anti-inflammatory action. Including the following foods in your diet could help to decrease inflammation; however, as some of them can help to thin the blood, they should not be eaten by patients on blood thinning medication or on prescribed anti-inflammatories.

Oils

Extra virgin Olive oil and canola oil both have high levels of vitamin E and omega oils that can be helpful in reducing inflammation. These oils are also believed to be beneficial to the heart.

Nuts and Seeds

Nuts and seeds are high in omega 6 fatty acids. Omega 6 has to be obtained through the diet or from supplementation, as it cannot be produced by the body.

Omega 6 has been found to help reduce nerve pain in patients with diabetic neuropathy.

Vegetables

Kale, broccoli, cauliflower, cabbage and sprouts can have powerful anti—inflammatory properties.

Fresh Fish

Any fresh fish will be high in omega oils, which are known to help beat inflammation. In addition to reducing inflammation, fresh fish is beneficial for the heart and the joints.

A diet rich in sugar, trans fats, meat, simple sugars and dairy foods can contribute to inflammation in the body, so consumption of these foods should be reduced.

Caffeine can also cause inflammation, as it will increase the cortisol levels in the body. High cortisol levels cause the body to feel stressed, and this process can lead to inflammation.

Chapter 7) Other Causes of Heel Pain

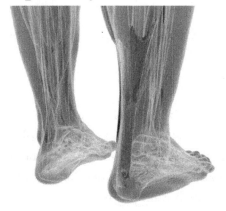

There can be many different reasons for heel pain. As explained at the beginning of the book, what makes tarsal tunnel syndrome different is the symptoms of nerve problems, such as burning sensations and electric shocks.

Detailed in this chapter are some of the other causes of heel pain and what you can do about them.

1) Achilles Tendonitis

Many people will experience heel pain when they have Achilles tendonitis. Tendonitis is often an overuse injury; it can be caused by excess pronation, wearing high heels, being overweight or poor biomechanics.

The Achilles is the strongest tendon in the body, but it is also extremely susceptible to inflammation and micro tears that can lead to Achilles tendonitis or tendinopathy.

Achilles tendonitis can eventually lead to tarsal tunnel syndrome if left untreated or allowed to worsen, so if you experience any

63

symptoms of Achilles tendonitis, then get them seen to straight away.

Chapter 6 offers a more detailed explanation of what to do, should Achilles tendonitis occur.

2) Plantar Fasciitis

The plantar tendon that runs along the bottom of the foot is often prone to inflammation. If left untreated, it can develop into plantar fasciitis, which can be difficult to treat; tarsal tunnel syndrome is often mistaken for this in its early stages and plantar fasciitis can cause burning sensations along the bottom of the foot.

The first stage of treatment is anti-inflammatories, rest and ice or warmth, whichever works best for the individual.

Next, you'll need to look at wearing supportive footwear or wearing insoles or heel pads to reduce the discomfort. If treated early enough, and if the causes of the inflammation are addressed, there is no need for anything more for conservative treatment and surgery wouldn't normally be considered.

3) Heel Fracture

The most common cause of a heel fracture is a fall, especially if it is from a height. The pain will be felt in the heel bone and patients will be unable to put their weight on the heel without pain.

The injury will need to be treated as soon as possible and surgery is often required to repair the fractured Calcaneal bone.

4) Heel Spurs

People often describe a heel spur as feeling like they have a stone in their shoe when they walk. The spur can cause a sharp pain in the heel of the foot when weight is put on it. Typically, the pain will be worse in the morning and patients will often experience a tightening in the calf area.

Heel spurs can often be a result of Achilles tendonitis or plantar fasciitis. People who pronate when they walk, people who overuse their muscles and people who just push themselves too hard can all be prone to this condition. If a deep, burning pain is felt in the heel after exercising, then book an appointment with your GP or a sports injury clinic and get your foot examined.

Topical anti-inflammatories, anti-inflammatory medication and ice are often the first courses of action. Sports massage, regular stretching and wearing a heel wedge or support can help to prevent this painful condition.

5) Ganglion

A ganglion can also cause heel pain. In addition, it can contribute to the symptoms of tarsal tunnel syndrome and an MRI scan will often show the ganglion in the heel. Ganglions can sometimes be visible on the outside of the foot. They are also common in the wrist area.

A ganglion is a cyst that fills with fluid and it will form in the joint or in the sheath of a tendon. Orthotics can be used to help heal the discomfort and if the cyst is severe then surgery to remove it will be discussed. However, sometimes the ganglion will just go away on its own, but they do often reoccur.

Various factors can contribute to the development of a ganglion. Biomechanics and wearing high heels can all be possible causes. If you have a ganglion then your doctor should investigate all possible causes of the development of the ganglion.

6) Bursitis

Bursitis is an inflammation of the bursa sac. This type of inflammation can affect the elbow and knees, but it is also relatively common in the ankle joints and heel.

It can be caused by overuse, and running is one of the common causes of this type of inflammation. Treatments for this condition include using anti-inflammatory medication to help reduce the pain and swelling; using an ice pack can also be useful.

People prone to bursitis need to make sure that they warm up and cool down before exercising and wear supportive sports shoes to avoid any excessive strain on the muscles of the feet.

Going for a biomechanical assessment would be a wise idea if this painful inflammation continues to be a problem, so suggestions can be made to find suitable orthotics to address any issues with the gait when running; a gait analysis would also be useful for patients with plantar fasciitis and Achilles tendonitis.

7) High Heels

Wearing high heels can contribute to heel pain due to the poor position the foot is held in. The plantar flexed position of the foot causes too much stress on the tendons, which can lead to conditions such as plantar fasciitis or Achilles problems.

If you absolutely must wear heels, make sure you wear an insole designed to take the stress off of the foot, make sure you stretch regularly to avoid the tendons getting too tight, and don't spent too long standing in high heels.

8) Short Achilles Tendon

A short Achilles tendon will cause pain in the heel region. The patient will also notice other symptoms, such as difficulty getting the heel on the ground or walking with their foot in a dropped position.

In the initial stages of treatment for a short tendon, doctors might advise wearing a heel pad to try and take the stress of the heel, but this can mean the tendon and calf will not have to stretch out as much and can cause the tendons in the lower leg to shorten even more.

Patients with a short Achilles tendon might also be sent to a physiotherapist to get exercises to try and lengthen the tendon. However, if the tendon is just too short, stretching won't be enough to elongate the Achilles adequately and surgery would be considered the best option.

A short tendon can also cause other aches and pains throughout the body; back pain is common in patients with short Achilles tendons.

9) Inflamed Heel Pad

The heel pad of the foot can become inflamed causing pain in this region. This can sometimes be caused by muscle wasting or atrophy.

For inflammation of the heel pad, anti-inflammatory medication will be the first course of action and patients might be advised to use ice to reduce any swelling.

Relieving the pain caused by inflammation of the heel pad will depend very much on the cause. If the patient has a muscle wasting condition and they have lost some of the protective padding on the heel, then it might be suggested that they wear something in the shoe to pad it out.

Supportive shoes that have a gel support in the heel region, such as the ones sold by Asics or New Balance, would be useful in this case as they provide the cushioning the foot needs.

Chapter 8) Tarsal Tunnel Syndrome and Carpal Tunnel Syndrome

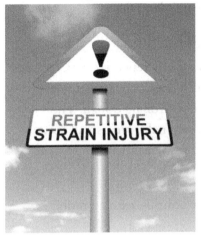

It can be quite common for patients with tarsal tunnel syndrome to also have carpal tunnel syndrome. There is some evidence to suggest that this isn't a coincidence, according to a study carried out in Italy.

The research found that these patients often had a narrow carpal tunnel, which could also mean that they had a narrow tarsal tunnel in the foot. This in turn could lead to a compression of both the median nerve and the tibial nerves, causing the symptoms of these two nerve entrapments.

1) Symptoms of Carpal Tunnel Syndrome

The symptoms of carpal tunnel syndrome include:

- Pain in the hands and fingers
- Pain in the wrists
- Feelings of electrical shocks
- Numbness in the hands
- Discomfort in the forearm and shoulders.

Patients might also develop muscle weakness due to the nerve compression and some might also find that their muscles begin to atrophy. Should this occur, there are several products on the market to help with problems with gripping and dexterity.

2) Causes of Carpal Tunnel Syndrome

Carpal Tunnel Syndrome is often caused by repetitive actions, such as typing or using a till. Bakers can also develop carpal tunnel syndrome due to the repetitive actions of rolling dough. The numbness some patients experience can make even small tasks difficult to manage if the symptoms aren't dealt with as soon as possible.

Patients with diabetes, low thyroid or arthritis are also more susceptible to this condition

3) Managing Carpal Tunnel Syndrome

Exercise balls are available to help keep the muscles strong and grip devices will help manage things, such as undoing lids and tins much easier.

Splints can be worn to reduce the stress on the hands and wrists when you are typing, or using a till, and breaking up repetitive actions by changing to do something else or stopping to stretch your hands and wrists out can be helpful. If you are suffering from carpal tunnel syndrome and decide to wear a split, then make sure that it is medically approved and that it fits properly or you risk making the symptoms worse if the splint doesn't provide adequate support.

Exercises can be done to help keep the hands mobile and to keep the muscles strong, if muscle loss and problems with dexterity become an issue. You'll find links to exercises in the resources chapter at the back of the book.

Patients with this condition could also benefit from seeing an occupational therapist. An occupational therapist can suggest ways to set up your work area to make it more ergonomically friendly, thus reducing stress and strain on the upper body and hands.

An occupational therapist can also suggest devices to make everyday tasks easier to manage. These services can be accessed through a GP, hospital physio or via social services, especially if you need help around the home.

Treatments for carpal tunnel syndrome tend to be on the conservative side, unless the symptoms become too severe, then surgery to release the compression in the median tendon will be discussed.

Otherwise, the main focus will be on medications such as anti-inflammatory drugs or steroids. Cortisone injections might also be used to help reduce pain and inflammation, but none of these medications are suitable for long term use and cortisone injections can cause the symptoms to become worse to begin with, before getting better.

Help should be sought at the first onset of symptoms, especially if you suffer from diabetes, low thyroid or arthritis. Don't allow the condition to get worse, as the longer it is left, the more difficult it is to manage.

Most of the time, no specific tests are needed to diagnose this condition. Once a GP has made a note of all of the symptoms, such as tingling and numbness, then the doctor is likely to ascertain that you have carpal tunnel syndrome. From there, a course of medication might be prescribed and you may be referred to a physiotherapist for exercises.

Chapter 9) Tarsal Tunnel Syndrome Private Care or Not

As I am from the UK, I can only explain the situation for private care in the UK. I assume, in the US, the situation is different.

Whether your treatment is undertaken by the NHS (National health Service in the UK) or a private hospital it will mainly consist of the same care options. The biggest difference will be the waiting times for an initial appointment.

If you choose to go private, the hospital will usually see you within a couple of days, but you'll have to get a referral letter from your GP first.

The cost of private care is often out of many people's reach, however, patients can ask to go to a private hospital – for a fee – to get the tests done and then ask for the results to be sent back to their own doctor so there won't be the costs of ongoing private appointments.

If the pain is severe, then getting a private referral can be a good idea if it eases your mind and gives you an answer as to what is causing your symptoms.

NHS waiting times will vary. It can often be up to four months for the first appointment with a neurologist and the waiting list for surgery – if it is required – will be much longer.

1) Physiotherapy for Tarsal Tunnel Syndrome

Depending on the area they live in, patients can self-refer to an NHS physio rather than waiting for a doctor to write a referral letter. If a GP suggests that seeing a physio would be beneficial, leaflets are available in surgeries that give contact details for the local physio clinic at the hospital. If self-referring, you'll be asked a set of questions about how your condition is affecting you; you might also be sent a questionnaire ahead of your first physio appointment asking some general questions about your health.

Due to the demands on the NHS, there can often be a waiting list for an appointment and it can take up to four months in some areas. Moreover, some NHS trusts limit patients to four sessions of therapy, which might not be enough if you have a chronic condition, but patients can go back to their doctor and ask for a new referral, and the process will start again.

After discussing your symptoms with you and reviewing the information on the questionnaire, the therapist will work with you to find some methods to better manage your condition. They might also give you a sheet of tailored exercises to do.

2) Private Physiotherapist Appointments

If you choose to go to a private hospital for physio, then a referral from your GP will still be required. However, getting an appointment is much easier and typically only takes a couple of days.

If you choose to go to a sports injury clinic, then there is no need for a referral, you can just choose the nearest one and make an appointment. If it is a case of trying to better manage your pain and keep mobile, then this is usually the easiest option.

With sports injury clinics, there are no limits to how many appointments you can have, and the staff can spend longer with you to help assess your condition. They can also work with you to help address any underlying condition that might be contributing to your tarsal tunnel syndrome. Sports injury clinics often stock insoles and can help teach you different taping methods if pronation or flat feet are contributing to your condition. They can also suggest managing your exercise routines differently, if overuse or tendonitis has caused the symptoms.

3) Surgery for Tarsal Tunnel Syndrome

The surgery offered via private hospitals will be the same that is provided by the NHS. However, patients going private won't have the long waiting lists to contend with.

The path to surgery is often a lengthy one; referral times to see a consultant can take up to six months, sometimes longer, depending on the area you live in. If, on your initial appointment, it is decided that surgery is necessary, then you'll be placed on a waiting list.

If it is not considered an emergency, then waiting times can be as long as 12-18 months, but this can sometimes be moved forward if there is a cancellation.

However, all courses of conservative treatment will be tried first, and it is only if none of these options relieve the symptoms that surgery will be considered an option.

As you might imagine, surgery via a private hospital is a much quicker process. Again, you'll need a doctor's referral for the first appointment and you can choose to see the doctor of your choice.

Patients can usually be seen within a few days. If your pain is severe and your symptoms are difficult to cope with, then exploring the options for private surgery is worthwhile.

4) Pain Management

If your pain has become chronic, and the medication you have been prescribed is not enough. Then a referral to a pain clinic should be considered. Pain clinics are assessable by going to your GP or consultant.

While the first appointment might take some time, the specialist will discuss how your pain affects your day to day life and how your symptoms affect the activities that you can do.

You'll be asked for information about the medication that you are already on and you might also have to undergo a brief examination.

As well as prescribing different medications to help with pain control, the staff can introduce you to a team of specialists that can help you cope better with your condition.

Some alternative therapies are available on the NHS and the one form of therapy often recommended by a pain clinic is acupuncture, as this has been proven to be an effective form of pain management for many individuals, especially when other methods have failed.

Acupuncture is usually made available as a short course of treatments and can also be effective in reducing the pain caused by muscle spasms.

The waiting lists for accessing acupuncture on the NHS are pretty long, and can sometimes take up to a year, as there is a strong demand for these services.

However, if you decide that this is a possible way forward in your treatment regimen, then it is a good idea to see a practitioner yourself. This form of complimentary therapy starts from around £35-£40 and depending on the severity of your condition, a ten week course might be necessary.

There are other effective methods of coping with pain naturally; you can read about these in chapter 12; in the back of the book you'll find details of where to find an acupuncturist.

Whether you go to an NHS hospital or a private hospital, there are ways of effectively managing your symptoms and making your life much more comfortable.

Some of the services can be hard to access and waiting times can sometimes seem too long, especially when you are in pain, but it is worth pursuing.

With the heavy demand placed on the NHS, some doctors can be reluctant to make the necessary referrals, but don't be put off by this either. Sometimes it is just a matter of trying a different approach or even an entirely different GP.

Private care might seem out of many people's reach, but often just a few appointments can be enough to help you get on top of the worst of the symptoms and help you find an effective management plan for your condition.

Whether or not you go private for your treatment, do seek a second opinion if surgery is suggested or if conservative treatments are found to be effective. By seeing another medical expert, you can often gain a new perspective on your condition and find new means of managing it.

Whichever path you choose, make sure that you know all of the various treatment options available to you and don't rule anything out that can help you cope with your tarsal tunnel syndrome.

Finding an effective form of therapy, whether it be through NHS or private means, will help you regain control over your condition and enable you to get your life back on track.

Chapter 10) Helping Yourself

Sometimes there is no quick answer to a medical problem. However, this book should have equipped you with enough knowledge to take some steps to help yourself.

Finding ways of effectively managing your condition is an empowering feeling and being proactive in your health care will help keep you feeling positive.

Here are some further steps you can take to help aid your recovery.

1) Join support groups

While it might not be possible to find a group near to you that offers support to patients with nerve pain, there are many to choose from on the Internet.

On these forums, you can ask questions that you might not have thought of asking your own GP or consultant, make queries about specific aspects of tarsal tunnel syndrome, and seek advice on how other people successfully manage their condition.

In the back of the book, there is a list of helpful associations and forums that will be useful if you decide you want to share your experiences with other people, or if you want to ask for advice yourself.

2) Mobilise and Exercise

If your tarsal tunnel syndrome makes you less active, then find some ways to keep mobile, as this will help to prevent muscle wasting, which could have a longer term effect on your mobility if it gets too serious.

77

As well as the exercises suggested earlier on in the book, find some ways of keeping yourself active. Exercises like Tai Chi, Chi Kung, and Qi Qong can all be beneficial for improved balance and circulation.

Yoga can be especially good for relaxing the muscles, thus preventing spasms. It can also aid balance and relaxation, as well as improve the circulation.

Try joining an exercise class that has been designed specifically for people with health issues or maybe use some exercise DVDs that have been created for people with limited mobility in mind.

However, don't begin an exercise programme without getting medical advice.

3) Take Control of your Pain

Whether you decide to take a prescribed medication or would prefer to take some natural alternatives to try to see how they work, then make sure you find a way to effectively manage your pain and any of the other associated symptoms of tarsal tunnel syndrome.

Chronic pain can lead to depression, and then it can become even more difficult to find a way to help yourself- so pain management needs to be a priority.

If the burning, tingling or electrical shock sensations cause you discomfort, then discuss taking a medication such as amitriptyline to help control this.

If you prefer natural methods, speak to the person responsible for your care first and seek a therapist who has an understanding of your condition.

4) Ask for Help

If mobility has become an issue and it is increasingly difficult to manage day to day activities in the same way that you used to, ask to see an occupational therapist.

An occupational therapist can suggest ideas to help you stay mobile around the house and they can also make a referral to a physiotherapist so you can get some helpful exercises to maintain mobility.

Occupational therapists can be accessed through your GP and through social services; some local councils have a form available online where you can request an appointment with an OT. They can also be accessed through the Job Centre, which is particularly helpful if your condition is making it difficult to stay in work, as they can refer you to a disability advisor to help address these issues.

5) Find out all you can

The more you learn about your condition, the easier it is to understand it and to find ways of coping. As new research or new techniques become available to help manage TTS, this information is often detailed online, so you can find out about new advances and how they might be applicable to you.

6) Get the care you need

Sometimes accessing some of the services is not easy, especially on an already overstrained NHS, but if you need help for your condition and you need means and methods of better coping with your TTS, then you are entitled to the care.

Some professionals aren't always great at making referrals when they are required and this can allow the condition to worsen and become more difficult to treat.

7) Find someone who understands

That can be harder than it seems at times, especially when you don't know anyone else with the same health problems, however, even just sharing how you feel with a close friend can make a whole lot of difference to how you approach things and can make you feel more positive about your situation.

Don't be afraid to ask for help or support when you need it and surround yourself with people that offer an understanding of your condition and how it affects you.

This is perhaps one of the most important things you can do to help yourself.

Chapter 11) Natural Pain Relief – Mind over Matter

Some people choose not to use conventional pain treatments and instead choose to try more natural methods. Detailed in this chapter are some ways that can help people deal with pain naturally, but please be aware that they might not be effective or suitable for everyone, and if you are in severe pain and need something to ease your discomfort quickly, then your best option is to find the right medication.

Studies have shown that controlling pain can sometimes be a case of mind over matter and by mastering some management techniques; it can become easier to cope with the pain from tarsal tunnel syndrome.

1) Distraction techniques

For many people, pain can often be worse when they are not occupied. Pain is nearly always worse at night, and one of the possible reasons for this is the fact that there is no distraction from it.

By getting involved in some other form of activity, preferably something that you find relaxing and enjoyable, you'll become less focused on the pain; if muscle spasm contributes to your pain levels, then the relaxation that comes about when you are immersed in something else and not focused on the pain or the feelings of tension, can help relax the spasms, which can somewhat reduce the pain.

2) Visualization

For some people, visualization can be a valuable aid to help with relaxation and chronic pain. You can either use your own imagination to create your own unique visualization, or follow one of the guided visualizations that can be found online.

Visualization typically begins with learning to relax and slowing your breathing and then picturing the image that you want to create in your mind. In could be one of sunshine and warmth healing the pain, or the ocean waves washing over you and taking away the discomfort. Use whichever technique works the best for you.

The best way to use this form of pain relief is to create an image that is the exact opposite of how you are feeling. For instance, if you feel like your feet are hot or burning, imagine them being plunged into a pool of cool, icy water and picture the water washing away the pain that you feel.

You'll find links in the resources chapter for guided visualizations.

3) Meditation

Meditation can be a useful tool to help gain control over pain and to create a calmer, more relaxed approach to how you manage your feelings of pain.

Studies have shown that using meditation techniques can also make people feel more accepting of their current situation and of the pain. Some meditations will also help the individual to begin to think differently about their suffering. There are several types of meditation to choose from when it comes to controlling pain.

Meditation is a gentle way to help reduce pain, and the techniques are simple to use. Meditation can also be useful to help counter everyday stresses and strains as well.

Mindfulness Meditation

As well as being useful to patients with chronic pain, mindfulness meditation can help to reduce stress levels and aid concentration and focus.

This type of meditation in gentle and easy to learn; CDs and DVDs are available if you are unable to find a class locally or just want to practice in your own time.

Breathing Meditation

Meditations that involve counting your breath can be helpful in pain management and at helping the mind and body to distress. The techniques don't take long to learn and beginners might find breathing meditation easier than some other forms, as it is simply to regain focus should they get distracted during the meditation process.

Breathing meditations are a useful tool for helping the body and mind to cope with every day stress and strains, and can help the body to unwind after a long day, thus reducing tension.

4) Hypnosis for Pain Management

Studies have shown that hypnosis can be effective for pain management. It has been proven to be an effective technique for managing the pain associated with arthritis and with disabilities, and for managing chronic or long lasting pain.

Hypnosis can also be used to reduce stress and anxiety, reduce tension and help to find ways to distract a patient from their pain.

Many books and CDs are available on this subject; you'll find details of them in the Further Reading section at the back of the book.

5) Cognitive Behavioral Therapy

Cognitive Behavioral Therapy, or CBT, has become increasing popular in recent years as a means for managing stress, anxiety and depression, but it can also be used to help manage pain effectively.

CBT can help a patient to control the negative emotions that are associated with their pain and then transform them into positive thoughts. Once the patient is thinking more positively, then they are better able to find ways to actively manage their condition.

Moreover, this form of therapy is excellent to help you set small goals that are achievable.

Several sessions of CBT will be required before a patient will start to feel better and be able to better manage their situation. CBT is available on the NHS in some areas of the UK and if a patient feels that they can benefit from this form of therapy, then they should ask their family doctor about this.

There have been issues about which type of patient CBT is suitable and when CBT will be considered a suitable course of therapy. You'll find a link to the guidelines in the sources chapter. However, if it is decided that you do not qualify for CBT treatment on the NHS then there are many books and CDs on the subject.

6) Deep Muscle Relaxation

This is best carried out last thing at night, especially if you find sleep difficult or if you are prone to cramps or stabbing pains during the night.

Deep muscle relaxation will allow the body to reduce tension, thus helping to combat some of the factors that can contribute to night time pain.

Deep relaxation involves relaxing each muscle one at a time, usually starting from the toes and the feet and up through the body. If during the process of deep relaxation any particular areas of tension are felt, then these areas can be concentrated on until they start to relax.

During the relaxation process, each muscle is tensed for approximately five seconds – sometimes longer – and then gently relaxed.

This is often best done after some other type of relaxation, such as yoga or meditation.

7) Biofeedback

Biofeedback can enable a person to learn how to re-educate their body to relax and to learn how to relax more deeply.

The technique involves using electronic assessment of the automatic functions of the body. This then allows an individual to gain control other the voluntary functions of the body.

Using biofeedback can help to reduce pain and muscle tension that has accumulated in the body. It can also help to reduce stress and blood pressure. It is also particularly good at helping a patient to gain control over parts of their body that are painful or that don't function as well as they should.

Other benefits of using this method include the ability to gain control over chronic pain, reduce painful muscle spasms and control the muscles.

Biofeedback machines are available, and they are easy to use, however, before using this kind of treatment, advice should be sought from a GP or consultant, to ensure that it is suitable as a form of therapy for your condition.

By using any of the above techniques, you can develop effective ways of pain management that can also be beneficial in other situations.

In Summary

In this book you will have found enough information to be able to manage tarsal tunnel syndrome effectively. You would have learnt how to differentiate the symptoms of the condition from other types of heel pain and the kinds of treatments and surgery available to relieve the problems that this type of compression neuropathy causes.

You'll also have found out about the natural remedies that are available, but these should only be used with the permission of the doctor and you would have learnt how to access services such as physiotherapy and occupational therapy, should they be required.

The successful management of this condition comes down to several steps:

- – Recognising and treating the symptoms
- – Pain management
- – Proper and timely diagnosis
- – Addressing the issues that lie behind TTS,
- – Exercise
- – Avoiding overuse of the muscles
- – Prevention

In this book, you should have all of the information you need to be able to work with your medical team and you will have learnt about the different avenues of treatment – both medical and alternative – that are available for you.

Sometimes it just comes down to trying various different methods until you find something that is right for you – and once you do – keep working with it.

In the following chapters you'll discover the support groups that are available for you, a suppliers' directory so you can purchase any of the products listed in this book, and a list of books for further reading.

Resources

If some of the links of these resources no longer work, just go to the main website and search for what you are looking for. Sometimes web masters do move pages to different locations on their web sites.

Exercises for Carpal Tunnel Syndrome:

The following video features three exercises for managing carpal tunnel syndrome.

http://www.youtube.com/watch?v=gTxQqu9USC4

This video features a yoga practice for those with carpal tunnel syndrome. They are also beneficial for patients who spend a lot of time at a desk.

http://www.youtube.com/watch?v=ztcfsNANTYg

The following video has exercises designed to strengthen the feet:

http://www.youtube.com/watch?v=moYSJBrPdHI&list=PLe0eeC6i5SzofdV1YHXa535CCTVyC4csN

And this video explains how to prevent pain in the heel:

http://www.youtube.com/watch?v=aAzpjU9NNQw

Chronic Pain advice

http://chronicpainsite.com/mb/?gclid=CKHFyILkoLsCFZGWtAodXA0A5g

Chronic Pain Visualization

http://www.howtocopewithpain.org/resources/relaxation-visualization-exercise.html

The Inner Health Studio offers a list of visualizations to choose from. They can be recorded for your own personal use, but they are copyrighted so they can't be sold on or used for any other commercial activity.

The site also has a podcast where listeners can get the latest visualizations.

http://www.innerhealthstudio.com/visualization-scripts.html

Chronic Pain Meditations

http://www.meditainment.com/pain-management/

http://www.youtube.com/watch?v=vW7y6qJMz5c

Recommended Guidelines for Pain Management for Adults:

http://www.britishpainsociety.org/book_pmp_main.pdf

Tarsal tunnel syndrome -emedicine

Emedicine has a useful overview of entrapment neuropathies:

http://emedicine.medscape.com/article/249784-overview

Forums

Forums are a great place to meet people who are suffering from the same problem as you. They offer an understanding community with other sufferers who are to share their experiences and help others.

They also provide a great opportunity for asking questions and getting the support you need. Listed below is a selection of nerve entrapment and pain management forums.

ABC Homeopathy Forum

This homeopathy forum has several discussions on the use of homeopathy for treating the symptoms of nerve compression neuropathies

If you don't see your questions answered, then feel free to post your own.

http://abchomeopathy.com/forum2.php/147010/

Bodywork Forum

The site has discussions on the difference between nerve compression, entrapment and impingement, as well as other topics.

http://www.bodyworkonline.com/forum/viewtopic.php?t=2327

Exchanges Pain Management Forum

Find useful information and strategies on successfully managing pain.

http://exchanges.webmd.com/pain-management-exchange/forum/index

Pain Support Forum

The Pain Support Forum was set up by Jan Sadler, MBE. She is the author of *Pain Relief Without Drugs;* the site is packed full of suggestions to help people manage pain. There is also a newsletter available.

http://www.painsupport.co.uk/index.asp

Suppliers' Directory

If some of the links of these resources no longer work, just go to the main website and search for what you are looking for. Sometimes web masters do move pages to different locations on their web sites.

Some of these products can be hard to obtain, so listed in this section of the suppliers' directory is a list of Internet retailers that are based in the UK, US, Australia and Canada.

If you prefer to buy products offline, then specialist sports' stores would be the best option for footwear and orthotics. However, a number of products in this category are only available from Internet sellers.

UK

Aircast A60 Ankle Support

Health and Care supply products designed to help manage disabilities and sports injury. The Aircast support will help to stop the foot from rolling over, so it is useful for people who pronate when they walk and have more pronation when they are active or tired.

They also supply products to relieve heel pressure.

http://www.healthandcare.co.uk/ankle-supports-braces/aircast-a60-ankle-support.html?gclid=CMnM1LH_o7sCFWgJwwodD3QAdw

Scholl Ortha Heel Insoles

The insoles can be bought from the Chiropdist.com. This product is suitable for people who wear shallow shoes and want something slim to fit inside them. The insole helps relieve heel pressure.

http://www.thechiropodist.com/product-scholl-orthaheel-regular-insoles.html

Swede O Tarsal

These can be a bit difficult to get hold of in the UK. The product is available from Amazon; however, the shipping can be very expensive. If you want to try and obtain one of these supports, it is probably best to contact the distributors or look for suppliers on eBay.

Healix care Controltec Insole

The Mobility Pit Stop supplies the Healix care Controltec insoles and they also have a range of other mobility aid products and daily living aids.

https://mobilitypitstop.com/0/2889/healix-care-controltec-insoles

Spenco Total Control

Physio Room supply a large range of Spenco products. The range includes insoles and heel cups to help relieve pain and protect the foot during exercise.

http://www.physioroom.com/brand.php?mid=281&affid=7&gclid=CNjys72zpLsCFUzHtAodxgMAGg

Sorbothane Sorbo-Pro Total Control

First Aid 4 Sports are one of the retailers of Sorborthane products. They also stock products for Achilles problems, and heel cups to help reduce heel pain, as well as many other sports care products.

http://www.firstaid4sport.co.uk/Sorbothane-Pro-Insoles-PSB92/

Silipos Malleolar Sleeve

These can be brought from DLT Podiatry.

http://www.dltpodiatry.co.uk/Gel-Sleeves-Silipos-Podopro/silipos-malleolar-sleeve.htm

Fs6 Compression Foot Sleeve

The compression sleeves can be ordered from Boots.com or from Amazon.

http://www.boots.com/en/FS6-Compression-Foot-Sleeve-S-M-sizes-4-8-_1285253/

Dr. Scholl's Insoles Tri-Comfort Orthotics

The orthotics can be ordered from eBay, Amazon, or direct from the manufacturers.

http://www.drscholls.com/Products/TriComfortregOrthotics

Pro-Tec Ankle Sleeve Support

The sleeve supports can be brought from Physioscience:

http://www.physioscienceuk.com/product/ankle/pro-tec-ankle-sleeve-support/

Power Ionics Compression supports

The supports are available on Amazon,

http://www.amazon.co.uk/Power-Ionics-Charcoal-Compression-236-BF001-Gi/dp/B00EP5B8MK

Or eBay:

http://www.amazon.co.uk/Power-Ionics-Charcoal-Compression-236-BF001-Gi/dp/B00EP5B8MK

Suppliers' Directory continued: Shoes, orthotics and compression stockings/socks

Australia

Swede 0- Tarsal

The brace is available from Australian Physiotherapy equipment in Australia. They also sell strapping products, tape, massage creams and lotions.

http://www.apemedical.com.au/shop/detail/swede-o-tarsal-lok/

Healix care Controltec Insole

The insoles can be difficult to find in Australia, but they can be bought from eBay.com.au site

Sorbothane Sorbo-Pro Total Control Insoles

Activ Instinct, an Australian-based store that offers sports products and supply these insoles.

http://www.activinstinct.com/au/running/athletic-supports/insoles/sorbothane-sorbo-pro-insole/

Fs6 Compression Foot Sleeve

In Australia, these can be purchased form a specialist store called Sole Integrity.

http://www.soleintegrity.com.au/brands/fs-6/fs-6-compression-foot-sleeve-pair

Scholl Ortha Heel Insoles

Scholl products can be obtained from the Walking Company.

http://www.thewalkingcompany.com.au/brand/scholl-orthaheel

Aircast A60 Ankle Brace

The braces can be bought from:

http://www.ausmedsupply.com.au/showProduct/Bracing/Foot+and+Ankle/81-02TXX/Aircast+A60+Ankle+Brace+Retail+Packaging

Dr. Scholl's Insoles Tri-Comfort Orthotics

Orthotics can be bought from:

http://www.ebay.com.au/itm/DR-SCHOLL-TRI-COMFORT-ORTHOTICS-SHOE-INSOLES-MEN-SIZE-8-12-BRAND-NEW-GET-RELIEF-/111020956184

Power Ionics Compression supports

These can be obtained via eBay.com.au.

http://www.ebay.com.au/itm/2pcs-Power-Ionics-Bamboo-Charcoal-Elastic-Compression-Wrist-Sleeve-Brace-Support-/150956972373

Suppliers' Directory continued: Shoes, orthotics and compression stockings/socks

United States and Canada

Spence Total Control Insoles

The insoles can be bought from feetrelief.com. They accept credit card payments, and products can be bought online, by phone, or by filling out a printed form and mailing the order direct to the address given on their website.

http://www.usmedical1.com/product.php?id_product=100

Compression Socks

Compression socks can be bought from:

http://www.footsourcemd.com/products/detail.dT/54

The site also has a selection of other productions to help manage foot pain and maintain foot health.

Swede 0- Tarsal

The Swede 0- Tarsal can be obtained from US Medical Supplies.

http://www.usmedicalsupplies.com/22815RUS-M.html

Healix care Controltec Insole

The insoles can be difficult to find in Australia, but they can be bought from the eBay.com.au site.

http://www.usmedical1.com/product.php?id_product=100

Spenco Total Control

These can be hard to obtain in Australia, however, a US-based company called The Insole Store ship internationally, so they can be obtained from there.

http://www.theinsolestore.com/spenco-polysorb-total-support-sandals.html

Sorbothane Sorbo-Pro Total Control

If there are difficulties obtaining the insoles in the US, then refer to the manufacturer's website for a list of suppliers or visit eBay.com.

http://www.sorbothane.co.uk/page9a55.html?section=22&sectionTitle=Buy+online

Silipos Malleolar Sleeve

Universal Medical supply the full range of Silipos products.

http://www.universalmedical.com.au/category53_2.htm

Fs6 Compression Foot Sleeve

They can be sourced direct from the manufacturers by visiting:

http://www.ingsource.com/

Scholl Ortha Heel Insoles

These can be bought from Amazon.com

http://www.amazon.com/Scholl-Orthaheel-Regular-Orthotic-Medium/dp/B003ASYE4C

Aircast A60 Ankle Brace

They are available from eBay.com, and they are less expensive than other retailers.

http://www.ebay.com/itm/AirCast-A60-Ankle-Brace-Support-Compression-Therapy-All-Sizes-New-/200783159891

Dr. Scholl's Insoles Tri-Comfort Orthotics

The orthotics can be ordered from Amazon.com.

http://www.amazon.com/Dr-Scholls-Tri-Comfort-Orthotic-Insoles/dp/B0000798CT

Pro-Tec Ankle Sleeve Support

They can be bought from:

http://www.legstherapy.com/braces-and-supports/pro-tec-ankle-sleeve-support.html

Power Ionics Compression supports

They can be bought from:

http://www.ebay.com/itm/Power-Ionics-Bamboo-Fiber-Blood-Circulation-Heat-Arthritis-Ankle-Brace-Support-/261144253128

Canada

The tarsal support brace can be bought from the official distributors in Canada and the US.

http://www.pattersonmedical.ca/app.aspx?cmd=searchResults&sk=swede-o

Healix care Controltec Insole

They are available from ebay.com. They can also be purchased from:

http://www.usmedical1.com/cms.php?id_cms=1

Spenco Insoles

In Canada, Spenco insoles can be purchased from well.ca.

http://well.ca/brand/spenco.html

Sorbothane Sorbo-Pro Total Control

If the product proves hard to find in Canada, then Amazon retails these insoles. If there is a problem with shipping to Canada, then refer to the manufacturer's website where they list their approved suppliers.

http://www.sorbothane.co.uk/page9a55.html?section=22&sectionTitle=Buy+online

Silipos Malleolar Sleeve

The compression sleeves can be obtained directly from the makers. They also sell gel socks, heel cups and wraps.

http://www.silipos.com/Products/Orthopedics/Sleeves-&-Wraps/Malleolar-Sleeve

Fs6 Compression Foot Sleeve

The foot sleeves are available from Shop To It:

http://www.shoptoit.ca/fs6-compression-foot-sleeve/35008663/

The store also sells many other useful dialing living aids.

Scholl Ortha Heel Insoles

These can be obtained from Amazon.com, if they prove difficult to find anywhere else.

http://www.amazon.com/Scholl-Orthaheel-Regular-Orthotic-Medium/dp/B003ASYE4C

Aircast A60 Ankle Brace

Braces can be obtained from:

http://clinicsuppliescanada.com/bracing-and-belts/ankle-brace-supports

Dr. Scholl's Insoles Tri-Comfort Orthotics

Visit http://www.drscholls.ca/en/products/tri-comfort-orthotics to order these products or to find suppliers in the Canada area.

Pro-Tec Ankle Sleeve Support

They can be bought from:

http://www.legstherapy.com/braces-and-supports/pro-tec-ankle-sleeve-support.html

Pro-Tec Ankle Sleeve Support

They can be bought from Amazon's Canadian site:

http://www.amazon.ca/Pro-Tec-Athletics-Force-Ankle-Sleeve/dp/B004TTLVI8

Power Ionics Compression supports

These can be ordered from eBay, if there is difficulty obtaining them anywhere else.

Compression stockings are available from:

http://www.daylong.co.uk/womens/compression-hosiery-style/

http://www.betterlifehealthcare.com/products.php?catID=1&subID=30&gclid=CNWpjc3Bj7sCFSoOwwodpXYAsw

http://www.betterlifehealthcare.com/products.php?catID=1&subID=30&gclid=CNWpjc3Bj7sCFSoOwwodpXYAsw

Tarsal Tunnel Compression socks can be bought from:

http://www.therapysocks.com/tarsal-tunnel-pain.html?gclid=COHVmsmdqLsCFQgOwwod904AyQ

Asics and New Balance shoes are available from sports stores and can be bought online.

Glossary

Plantar fasciitis

An inflammation of the plantar tendon in the foot.

Achilles tendon

The tendon that runs down the back of the leg and attaches the calf to the heel. It is the strongest tendon in the body.

Achilles tendonitis

An inflammation of the Achilles tendon.

Cross friction massage

Cross friction is a form of massage, most often used to help treat sports injury. It involves using moderation pressure.

Posterior tibial nerve

The posterior tibial nerve runs into the foot and has several branches. Finding which branches of nerves are affected is the most effective way of treating tarsal tunnel syndrome.

Deep peroneal nerve

The nerve is part of the peroneal nerve. The peroneal nerves branches out from the sciatic nerves.

Dorsiflexion

This describes the position of the foot when it is flexed towards the body.

Dorsiflexion eversion

A means of determining whether a patient has Tarsal Tunnel Syndrome.

Nerve conduction studies

Nerve conduction studies examine how well the nerves are firing and how fast.

EMG

An electromyogram will help diagnose nerve problems, such as tarsal and carpal tunnel syndrome.

MRI

An MRI scan creates internal imageries of the structures of the body.

Etiology

Etiology explores the reason or causes behind a disease or condition.

Eversion

Refers to the foot pointing outwards when a person walks.

Physiotherapist

Physiotherapist's help to improve and maintain mobility and suggest exercises and massage techniques.

Aromatherapy

A form of therapy using the aroma of essential oils to help heal the mind and body

Osteopathy

A gentle, hands on technique to help mobilise the body and heal aches and pains.

Sports massage

A form of massage to help the body prepare for sports and to help the muscles relax and recover afterwards.

Trigger point massage

When touched, trigger points will cause pain in the body. Using massage can help to relieve this discomfort

Orthobionomy

Uses gentle manipulation and movement techniques.

Neuromuscular massage

This type of massage can help to release deep seated tender points that can trigger pain in the body

Chiropractor

A gentle manipulation of the body to reduce pain and ease movement.

Bone spurs

These form along joints and are formed from bone.

Hypothyroidism

A person with low levels of thyroid will be described as having hypothyroidism.

Low thyroid

Low levels of the hormone thyroxine, which is produced by the thyroid gland.

Diabetes

An inability of the islet cells of the pancreas to produce insulin.

Glucose levels

The measure of glucose in the blood stream commonly known as blood sugar.

Sources

Medial tarsal tunnel syndrome: a review.

http://www.ncbi.nlm.nih.gov/pubmed/18806381

Kushner S, Reid DC.

The dorsiflexion-eversion test for diagnosis of tarsal tunnel syndrome.

Kinoshita M, Okuda R, Morikawa J, Jotoku T, Abe M.

Source

Department of Orthopedic Surgery, Osaka Medical College, 2-7 Daigaku-machi, Takatsuki City, Osaka 569-8686, Japan

http://www.ncbi.nlm.nih.gov/pubmed/11741063

Usefulness of electrodiagnostic techniques in the evaluation of suspected tarsal tunnel syndrome: an evidence-based review.

http://www.ncbi.nlm.nih.gov/pubmed/9850949

Electrophysiological evidence of a relationship between idiopathic carpal and tarsal tunnel syndromes.

Mondelli M, Cioni R.

Source

EMG Service ASL 7, Siena, Italy.

http://www.sciencedirect.com/science/article/pii/S20905068 1200084X

Tarsal tunnel syndrome in patients with rheumatoid arthritis, electrophysiological and ultrasound study

http://www.ncbi.nlm.nih.gov/pubmed/16003732

Further Reading

The Layman's Guide to Foot and Heel Pain by Les Bailey

The Physiotherapist by Kenyon, Karen and Kenyon, Jonathan

15 Minutes To Happy Feet - Self Treatment Guide To Plantar Fasciitis by Rewick, Todd

The Foot Book: A Complete Guide to Healthy Feet (A Johns Hopkins Press Health Book) by Rose, Jonathan D. and Martorana, Vincent J.

Heel Pain by D.P.M. Stephen L. Barrett

Every Woman's Guide to Foot Pain by Bowman, Katy

Acupressure: How to cure common ailments the natural way by Michael Reed Gach

Fixing Your Feet by Vonhof, John

Deep Tissue Massage: A Visual Guide to Techniques by Riggs, Art and Myers, Thomas W

DVDs

Home Physio - Treat Your Own Leg Pain

Stott Pilates: Pain Free Posture

Yoga for Back Pain - Radha Yadav

Am/Pm Stretch for Health

Stretch and Joint Mobility Therapy, with Annette Fletcher: Body flexibility training to reduce joint stiffness, Stretching instruction

Acknowledgements

Special thanks to Mary Aspinwall for her contribution to the book.

Big thank you to my family for supporting me in whatever I do.

Index

CPSIA information can be obtained at www.ICGtesting.com
Printed in the USA
LVOW04s1116240814

400662LV00016B/809/P